Logbook for
Foundation
Course

for **MBBS Students**

Student's Name: _____

Roll No.: _____   Year/Session: _____

University Roll No.: _____   Name of the Course: _____

Name of the Institution: _____

This is to certify that this is a bonafide practical work done by _____
during the year 20____ – 20____. His/her work is complete | incomplete | excellent | satisfactory | good | fair.

_____   _____

Signature of Staff in-charge   Signature of Professor & HOD

Submitted for University Examination in the year _____

Examiners: _____

Logbook for Foundation Course

for MBBS Students

Niket Verma MBBS, MD (General Medicine)
Assistant Professor
Department of General Medicine
Army College of Medical Sciences
Delhi Cantt.
New Delhi

Poonam Agrawal MBBS, MD (Biochemistry)
Professor
Department of Biochemistry
Dr. Baba Saheb Ambedkar Medical College and Hospital
Rohini
New Delhi

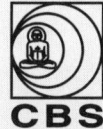

CBS

CBS Publishers & Distributors Pvt Ltd

New Delhi • Bengaluru • Chennai • Kochi • Kolkata • Mumbai
Bhopal • Bhubaneswar • Hyderabad • Jharkhand • Nagpur • Patna • Pune
• Uttarakhand • Dhaka (Bangladesh) • Kathmandu (Nepal)

Logbook for

Foundation Course

for **MBBS Students**

ISBN: 978-93-89261-77-6

Copyright © Authors and Publisher

First Edition: 2020

Published by Satish Kumar Jain and produced by Varun Jain for

CBS Publishers & Distributors Pvt Ltd

4819/XI Prahlad Street, 24 Ansari Road, Daryaganj, New Delhi 110 002, India.
Ph: 23289259, 23266861, 23266867   Website: www.cbspd.com
Fax: 011-23243014   e-mail: delhi@cbspd.com; cbspubs@airtelmail.in.
Corporate Office: 204 FIE, Industrial Area, Patparganj, Delhi 110 092

Ph: 4934 4934   Fax: 4934 4935   e-mail: publishing@cbspd.com; publicity@cbspd.com

Branches

- **Bengaluru:** Seema House 2975, 17th Cross, K.R. Road,
  Banasankari 2nd Stage, Bengaluru 560 070, Karnataka
  Ph: +91-80-26771678/79   Fax: +91-80-26771680   e-mail: bangalore@cbspd.com
- **Chennai:** 7, Subbaraya Street, Shenoy Nagar, Chennai 600 030, Tamil Nadu
  Ph: +91-44-26680620, 26681266   Fax: +91-44-42032115   e-mail: chennai@cbspd.com
- **Kochi:** 42/1325, 1326, Power House Road, Opposite KSEB Power House,
  Ernakulam 682 018, Kochi, Kerala
  Ph: +91-484-4059061-65   Fax: +91-484-4059065   e-mail: kochi@cbspd.com
- **Kolkata:** 6/B, Ground Floor, Rameswar Shaw Road, Kolkata-700 014, West Bengal
  Ph: +91-33-22891126, 22891127, 22891128   e-mail: kolkata@cbspd.com
- **Mumbai:** 83-C, Dr E Moses Road, Worli, Mumbai-400018, Maharashtra
  Ph: +91-22-24902340/41   Fax: +91-22-24902342   e-mail: mumbai@cbspd.com

Representatives

- **Bhopal**   0-8319310552
- **Nagpur**   0-9421945513
- **Dhaka (Bangladesh)**   01912-003485
- **Bhubaneswar**   0-9911037372
- **Patna**   0-9334159340
- **Kathmandu (Nepal)**   977-9818742655
- **Hyderabad**   0-9885175004
- **Pune**   0-9623451994
- **Jharkhand**   0-9811541605
- **Uttarakhand**   0-9716462459

Printed at Glorious Printers, Daryaganj, Delhi, India

Preface

Dear students

Congratulations on your selection into MBBS and welcome to the world of medicine !!

We share your excitement as you enter college, full of hope and confidence. As you are aware, there have been some changes in the existing system of medical education in our country. Competency Based Medical Education (CBME), which is being implemented from this year onwards, aims to make you competent Indian Medical Graduates at the end of your undergraduate training.

The new system focuses on small group teaching–learning, self-directed learning and early clinical exposure, among other things. Your curriculum has been divided into competencies. Each teaching–learning session will have certain learning objectives and will help you in attaining these competencies. As we all are living in the 'Information Age', there is increased emphasis on using information-technology enabled classrooms, skills laboratories and e-learning. There is renewed emphasis on the teaching (and learning !!) of soft skills, something that will help you in becoming not only better doctors, but also better human beings. Later during your training, you will also be taking up two electives of your choice, something that will help expand your horizons beyond the traditional boundaries of medicine.

Under the new system, the first month of MBBS is exclusively devoted to the 'Foundation Course'. The Foundation Course spans a total of 175 hours in which 30 hours are allotted for Orientation, 35 hours for Skills Modules, 8 hours for Field Visits, 40 hours for Professional Development including Ethics, 40 hours for Language and Computer Skills and 22 hours for Sports and Extracurricular Activities. The Foundation Course aims to introduce you to the medical profession and the role of a doctor in society.

During the next month you will get a chance to visit the various departments in your college and meet the faculty members, visit the hospital and community and primary health centres and understand the work of a healthcare team which includes doctors and allied healthcare staff and get an insight into the alternative health systems in our country. You will be introduced to first-aid, the importance of handwashing and the concept of biosafety. You will also learn about professionalism and ethics in medicine and the consequences of unprofessional and unethical behaviour. During the Foundation Course, you will get a chance to hone your language and computer skills and learn about time and stress management. In between all these sessions, there will be ample breaks and you will also be able to indulge in your favourite sports and extracurricular hobbies or learn new ones with your batchmates. All in all, it promises to be a very interesting month and we are sure you will enjoy every session. Remember, a strong foundation is the prerequisite to a strong building and many of the concepts and skills you learn during this month will help you face difficult situations and crises that you may encounter during your career as a medical professional.

This Logbook allows you to maintain a record of all the sessions conducted during the Foundation Course. This will help build your writing skills and allow you to reflect on what you have learnt in each session. Additionally, it will also serve as a nostalgic reminder of the wonderful first few days you spent in medical college.

Happy Learning !!

Niket Verma
Poonam Agrawal

Contents

Orientation

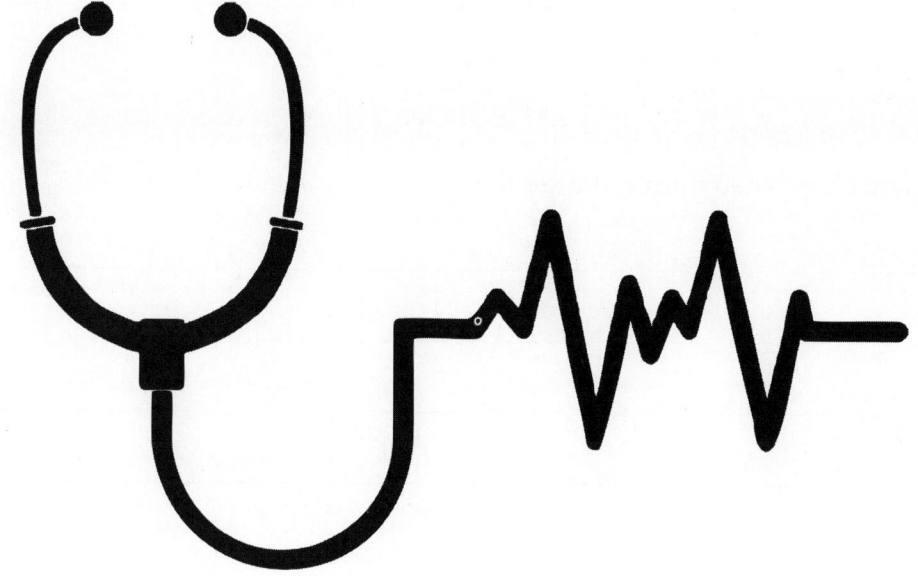

Orientation: Session 1

Name of the session: _____

Name of the faculty member(s): _____

Date:_____   Time: _____   Duration:_____

Learning objective(s) of the session:

1. _____   2. _____

3. _____   4. _____

Teaching learning method(s):_____

REFLECTION

A. Please describe what happened during the session:

_____

_____

_____

_____

B. What did you learn from the session?

_____

_____

_____

_____

C. How will it help you become a better doctor in the future?

_____

_____

_____

_____

Orientation: Session 2

Name of the session: _____

Name of the faculty member(s): _____

Date:_____   Time: _____   Duration:_____

Learning objective(s) of the session:

1. _____   2. _____

3. _____   4. _____

Teaching learning method(s):_____

REFLECTION

A. Please describe what happened during the session:

_____

_____

_____

_____

B. What did you learn from the session?

_____

_____

_____

_____

C. How will it help you become a better doctor in the future?

_____

_____

_____

_____

Orientation: Session 3

Name of the session: _____

Name of the faculty member(s): _____

Date:_____   Time: _____   Duration:_____

Learning objective(s) of the session:

1. _____   2. _____

3. _____   4. _____

Teaching learning method(s):_____

REFLECTION

A. Please describe what happened during the session:

_____

_____

_____

_____

B. What did you learn from the session?

_____

_____

_____

_____

C. How will it help you become a better doctor in the future?

_____

_____

_____

Orientation: Session 4

Name of the session: _____

Name of the faculty member(s): _____

Date:_____   Time: _____   Duration:_____

Learning objective(s) of the session:

1. _____   2. _____

3. _____   4. _____

Teaching learning method(s):_____

REFLECTION

A. Please describe what happened during the session:

_____

_____

_____

_____

B. What did you learn from the session?

_____

_____

_____

_____

C. How will it help you become a better doctor in the future?

_____

_____

_____

_____

Orientation: Session 5

Name of the session: _____

Name of the faculty member(s): _____

Date:_____   Time: _____   Duration:_____

Learning objective(s) of the session:

1. _____   2. _____

3. _____   4. _____

Teaching learning method(s):_____

REFLECTION

A. Please describe what happened during the session:

_____

_____

_____

_____

B. What did you learn from the session?

_____

_____

_____

_____

C. How will it help you become a better doctor in the future?

_____

_____

_____

Orientation: Session 6

Name of the session: _____

Name of the faculty member(s): _____

Date: _____   **Time:** _____   **Duration:** _____

Learning objective(s) of the session:

1. _____   2. _____

3. _____   4. _____

Teaching learning method(s): _____

REFLECTION

A. Please describe what happened during the session:

_____

_____

_____

_____

B. What did you learn from the session?

_____

_____

_____

_____

C. How will it help you become a better doctor in the future?

_____

_____

_____

_____

Orientation: Session 7

Name of the session: _____

Name of the faculty member(s): _____

Date: _____   Time: _____   Duration: _____

Learning objective(s) of the session:

1. _____   2. _____

3. _____   4. _____

Teaching learning method(s): _____

REFLECTION

A. Please describe what happened during the session:

_____

_____

_____

_____

B. What did you learn from the session?

_____

_____

_____

_____

C. How will it help you become a better doctor in the future?

_____

_____

_____

Orientation: Session 8

Name of the session: _____ __

Name of the faculty member(s): _____

Date:_____   Time:_____   Duration:_____

Learning objective(s) of the session:

1. _____   2. _____

3. _____   4. _____

Teaching learning method(s):_____

REFLECTION

A. Please describe what happened during the session:

_____

_____

_____

_____

B. What did you learn from the session?

_____

_____

_____

_____

C. How will it help you become a better doctor in the future?

_____

_____

_____

_____

Orientation: Session 9

Name of the session: _____

Name of the faculty member(s): _____

Date: _____   Time: _____   Duration: _____

Learning objective(s) of the session:

1. _____   2. _____

3. _____   4. _____

Teaching learning method(s): _____

REFLECTION

A. Please describe what happened during the session:

_____

_____

_____

_____

B. What did you learn from the session?

_____

_____

_____

_____

C. How will it help you become a better doctor in the future?

_____

_____

_____

_____

Orientation: Session 10

Name of the session: _____

Name of the faculty member(s): _____

Date:_____   Time:_____   Duration:_____

Learning objective(s) of the session:

1. _____   2. _____

3. _____   4. _____

Teaching learning method(s):_____

REFLECTION

A. Please describe what happened during the session:

_____

_____

_____

_____

B. What did you learn from the session?

_____

_____

_____

_____

C. How will it help you become a better doctor in the future?

_____

_____

_____

Orientation: Session 11

Name of the session: _____

Name of the faculty member(s): _____

Date: _____ Time: _____ Duration: _____

Learning objective(s) of the session:

1. _____ 2. _____

3. _____ 4. _____

Teaching learning method(s): _____

REFLECTION

A. Please describe what happened during the session:

_____

_____

_____

_____

B. What did you learn from the session?

_____

_____

_____

_____

C. How will it help you become a better doctor in the future?

_____

_____

_____

_____

Orientation: Session 12

Name of the session: _____

Name of the faculty member(s): _____

Date: _____   Time: _____   Duration: _____

Learning objective(s) of the session:

1. _____   2. _____

3. _____   4. _____

Teaching learning method(s): _____

REFLECTION

A. Please describe what happened during the session:

_____

_____

_____

_____

B. What did you learn from the session?

_____

_____

_____

_____

C. How will it help you become a better doctor in the future?

_____

_____

_____

_____

Orientation: Session 13

Name of the session: _____

Name of the faculty member(s): _____

Date:_____   Time: _____   Duration:_____

Learning objective(s) of the session:

1. _____   2. _____

3. _____   4. _____

Teaching learning method(s):_____

REFLECTION

A. Please describe what happened during the session:

_____

_____

_____

_____

B. What did you learn from the session?

_____

_____

_____

_____

C. How will it help you become a better doctor in the future?

_____

_____

_____

_____

Orientation: Session 14

Name of the session: _____

Name of the faculty member(s): _____

Date:_____ Time: _____ Duration:_____

Learning objective(s) of the session:

1. _____ 2. _____

3. _____ 4. _____

Teaching learning method(s):_____

REFLECTION

A. Please describe what happened during the session:

_____

_____

_____

_____

B. What did you learn from the session?

_____

_____

_____

_____

C. How will it help you become a better doctor in the future?

_____

_____

_____

_____

Orientation: Session 15

Name of the session: _____

Name of the faculty member(s): _____

Date:_____ Time: _____ Duration:_____

Learning objective(s) of the session:

1. _____   2. _____

3. _____   4. _____

Teaching learning method(s):_____

REFLECTION

A. Please describe what happened during the session:

_____

_____

_____

_____

B. What did you learn from the session?

_____

_____

_____

_____

C. How will it help you become a better doctor in the future?

_____

_____

_____

Orientation: Session 16

Name of the session: _____

Name of the faculty member(s): _____

Date:_____   Time: _____   Duration:_____

Learning objective(s) of the session:

1. _____   2. _____

3. _____   4. _____

Teaching learning method(s): _____

REFLECTION

A. Please describe what happened during the session:

_____

_____

_____

_____

B. What did you learn from the session?

_____

_____

_____

_____

C. How will it help you become a better doctor in the future?

_____

_____

_____

Orientation: Session 17

Name of the session: _____

Name of the faculty member(s): _____

Date:_____   Time: _____   Duration:_____

Learning objective(s) of the session:

1. _____   2. _____

3. _____   4. _____

Teaching learning method(s):_____

REFLECTION

A. Please describe what happened during the session:

_____

_____

_____

_____

B. What did you learn from the session?

_____

_____

_____

_____

C. How will it help you become a better doctor in the future?

_____

_____

_____

Orientation: Session 18

Name of the session: _____

Name of the faculty member(s): _____

Date: _____   **Time:** _____   **Duration:** _____

Learning objective(s) of the session:

1. _____   2. _____

3. _____   4. _____

Teaching learning method(s): _____

REFLECTION

A. Please describe what happened during the session:

_____

_____

_____

_____

B. What did you learn from the session?

_____

_____

_____

_____

C. How will it help you become a better doctor in the future?

_____

_____

_____

_____

Orientation: Session 19

Name of the session: _____

Name of the faculty member(s): _____

Date:_____   Time:_____   Duration:_____

Learning objective(s) of the session:

1. _____   2. _____

3. _____   4. _____

Teaching learning method(s):_____

REFLECTION

A. Please describe what happened during the session:

_____

_____

_____

_____

B. What did you learn from the session?

_____

_____

_____

_____

C. How will it help you become a better doctor in the future?

_____

_____

_____

Orientation: Session 20

Name of the session: _____

Name of the faculty member(s): _____

Date:_____   Time: _____   Duration:_____

Learning objective(s) of the session:

1. _____   2. _____

3. _____   4. _____

Teaching learning method(s):_____

REFLECTION

A. Please describe what happened during the session:

_____

_____

_____

_____

B. What did you learn from the session?

_____

_____

_____

_____

C. How will it help you become a better doctor in the future?

_____

_____

_____

_____

Orientation: Session 21

Name of the session: _____

Name of the faculty member(s): _____

Date:_____   Time: _____   Duration:_____

Learning objective(s) of the session:

1. _____   2. _____

3. _____   4. _____

Teaching learning method(s):_____

REFLECTION

A. Please describe what happened during the session:

_____

_____

_____

_____

B. What did you learn from the session?

_____

_____

_____

_____

C. How will it help you become a better doctor in the future?

_____

_____

_____

_____

Orientation: Session 22

Name of the session: _____

Name of the faculty member(s): _____

Date:_____   Time:_____   Duration:_____

Learning objective(s) of the session:

1. _____   2. _____

3. _____   4. _____

Teaching learning method(s):_____

REFLECTION

A. Please describe what happened during the session:

_____

_____

_____

_____

B. What did you learn from the session?

_____

_____

_____

_____

C. How will it help you become a better doctor in the future?

_____

_____

_____

_____

Orientation: Session 23

Name of the session: _____

Name of the faculty member(s): _____

Date:_____   Time:_____   Duration:_____

Learning objective(s) of the session:

1. _____   2. _____

3. _____   4. _____

Teaching learning method(s): _____

REFLECTION

A. Please describe what happened during the session:

_____

_____

_____

_____

B. What did you learn from the session?

_____

_____

_____

_____

C. How will it help you become a better doctor in the future?

_____

_____

_____

_____

Orientation: Session 24

Name of the session: _____

Name of the faculty member(s): _____

Date:_____   Time: _____   Duration:_____

Learning objective(s) of the session:

1. _____   2. _____

3. _____   4. _____

Teaching learning method(s):_____

REFLECTION

A. Please describe what happened during the session:

_____

_____

_____

_____

B. What did you learn from the session?

_____

_____

_____

_____

C. How will it help you become a better doctor in the future?

_____

_____

_____

_____

Orientation: Session 25

Name of the session: _____

Name of the faculty member(s): _____

Date:_____   Time: _____   Duration:_____

Learning objective(s) of the session:

1. _____   2. _____

3. _____   4. _____

Teaching learning method(s):_____

REFLECTION

A. Please describe what happened during the session:

_____

_____

_____

_____

B. What did you learn from the session?

_____

_____

_____

_____

C. How will it help you become a better doctor in the future?

_____

_____

_____

Orientation: Session 26

Name of the session: _____

Name of the faculty member(s): _____

Date:_____   Time: _____   Duration:_____

Learning objective(s) of the session:

1. _____   2. _____

3. _____   4. _____

Teaching learning method(s):_____

REFLECTION

A. Please describe what happened during the session:

_____

_____

_____

_____

B. What did you learn from the session?

_____

_____

_____

C. How will it help you become a better doctor in the future?

_____

_____

_____

Orientation: Session 27

Name of the session: _____

Name of the faculty member(s): _____

Date:_____   Time: _____   Duration:_____

Learning objective(s) of the session:

1. _____   2. _____

3. _____   4. _____

Teaching learning method(s): _____

REFLECTION

A. Please describe what happened during the session:

_____

_____

_____

_____

B. What did you learn from the session?

_____

_____

_____

_____

C. How will it help you become a better doctor in the future?

_____

_____

_____

_____

Orientation: Session 28

Name of the session: _____

Name of the faculty member(s): _____

Date:_____   Time: _____   Duration:_____

Learning objective(s) of the session:

1. _____   2. _____

3. _____   4. _____

Teaching learning method(s):_____

REFLECTION

A. Please describe what happened during the session:

_____

_____

_____

_____

B. What did you learn from the session?

_____

_____

_____

_____

C. How will it help you become a better doctor in the future?

_____

_____

_____

_____

Orientation: Session 29

Name of the session: _____

Name of the faculty member(s): _____

Date: _____   Time: _____   Duration: _____

Learning objective(s) of the session:

1. _____   2. _____

3. _____   4. _____

Teaching learning method(s): _____

REFLECTION

A. Please describe what happened during the session:

_____

_____

_____

_____

B. What did you learn from the session?

_____

_____

_____

_____

C. How will it help you become a better doctor in the future?

_____

_____

_____

_____

Orientation: Session 30

Name of the session: _____

Name of the faculty member(s): _____

Date: _____   **Time:** _____   **Duration:** _____

Learning objective(s) of the session:

1. _____   2. _____

3. _____   4. _____

Teaching learning method(s): _____

REFLECTION

A. Please describe what happened during the session:

_____

_____

_____

_____

B. What did you learn from the session?

_____

_____

_____

_____

C. How will it help you become a better doctor in the future?

_____

_____

_____

_____

Skills Module

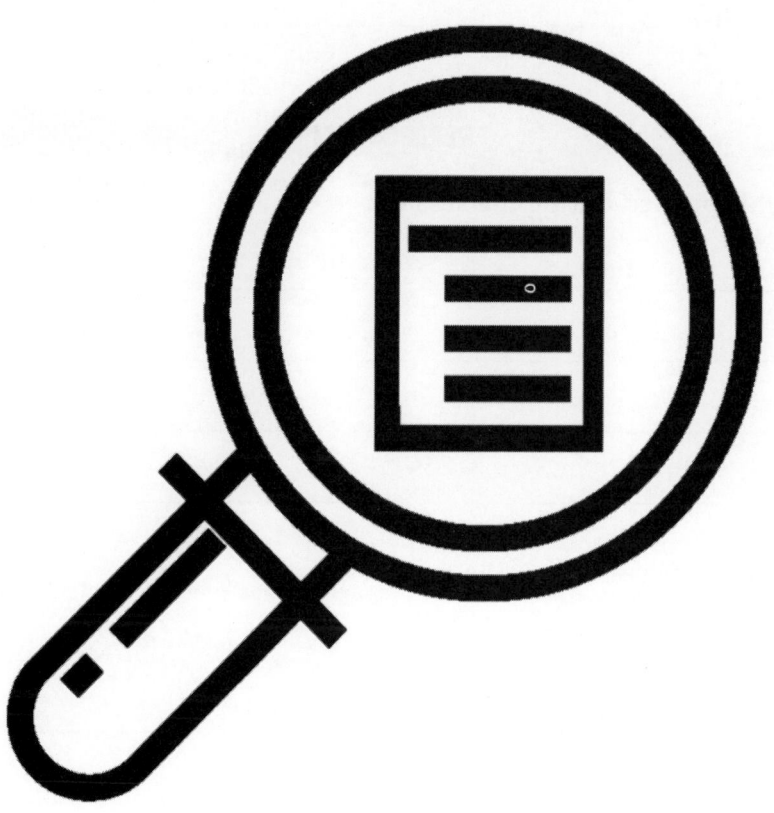

Skills Module: Session 1

Name of the session: _____

Name of the faculty member(s): _____

Date:_____   Time: _____   Duration:_____

Learning objective(s) of the session:

1. _____   2. _____

3. _____   4. _____

Teaching learning method(s):_____

REFLECTION

A. Please describe what happened during the session:

_____

_____

_____

_____

B. What did you learn from the session?

_____

_____

_____

_____

C. How will it help you become a better doctor in the future?

_____

_____

_____

_____

Skills Module: Session 2

Name of the session: _____

Name of the faculty member(s): _____

Date:_____   Time: _____   Duration:_____

Learning objective(s) of the session:

1. _____   2. _____

3. _____   4. _____

Teaching learning method(s):_____

REFLECTION

A. Please describe what happened during the session:

_____

_____

_____

_____

B. What did you learn from the session?

_____

_____

_____

_____

C. How will it help you become a better doctor in the future?

_____

_____

_____

Skills Module: Session 3

Name of the session: _____

Name of the faculty member(s): _____

Date: _____   Time: _____   Duration: _____

Learning objective(s) of the session:

1. _____   2. _____

3. _____   4. _____

Teaching learning method(s): _____

REFLECTION

A. Please describe what happened during the session:

_____

_____

_____

_____

B. What did you learn from the session?

_____

_____

_____

_____

C. How will it help you become a better doctor in the future?

_____

_____

_____

_____

Skills Module: Session 4

Name of the session: _____

Name of the faculty member(s): _____

Date: _____   Time: _____   Duration: _____

Learning objective(s) of the session:

1. _____   2. _____

3. _____   4. _____

Teaching learning method(s): _____

REFLECTION

A. Please describe what happened during the session:

_____

_____

_____

_____

B. What did you learn from the session?

_____

_____

_____

_____

C. How will it help you become a better doctor in the future?

_____

_____

_____

_____

Skills Module: Session 5

Name of the session: _____

Name of the faculty member(s): _____

Date:_____   Time: _____   Duration:_____

Learning objective(s) of the session:

1. _____   2. _____

3. _____   4. _____

Teaching learning method(s):_____

REFLECTION

A. Please describe what happened during the session:

_____

_____

_____

_____

B. What did you learn from the session?

_____

_____

_____

_____

C. How will it help you become a better doctor in the future?

_____

_____

_____

Skills Module: Session 6

Name of the session: _____

Name of the faculty member(s): _____

Date:_____   Time: _____   Duration:_____

Learning objective(s) of the session:

1. _____   2. _____

3. _____   4. _____

Teaching learning method(s):_____

REFLECTION

A. Please describe what happened during the session:

_____

_____

_____

_____

B. What did you learn from the session?

_____

_____

_____

_____

C. How will it help you become a better doctor in the future?

_____

_____

_____

Skills Module: Session 7

Name of the session: _____

Name of the faculty member(s): _____

Date: _____   Time: _____   Duration: _____

Learning objective(s) of the session:

1. _____   2. _____

3. _____   4. _____

Teaching learning method(s): _____

REFLECTION

A. Please describe what happened during the session:

_____

_____

_____

_____

B. What did you learn from the session?

_____

_____

_____

_____

C. How will it help you become a better doctor in the future?

_____

_____

_____

Skills Module: Session 8

Name of the session: _____

Name of the faculty member(s): _____

Date:_____ Time: _____ Duration:_____

Learning objective(s) of the session:

1. _____ 2. _____

3. _____ 4. _____

Teaching learning method(s):_____

REFLECTION

A. Please describe what happened during the session:

_____

_____

_____

_____

B. What did you learn from the session?

_____

_____

_____

_____

C. How will it help you become a better doctor in the future?

_____

_____

_____

Skills Module: Session 9

Name of the session: _____

Name of the faculty member(s): _____

Date: _____ Time: _____ Duration: _____

Learning objective(s) of the session:

1. _____ 2. _____

3. _____ 4. _____

Teaching learning method(s): _____

REFLECTION

A. Please describe what happened during the session:

_____

_____

_____

_____

B. What did you learn from the session?

_____

_____

_____

_____

C. How will it help you become a better doctor in the future?

_____

_____

_____

Skills Module: Session 10

Name of the session: _____

Name of the faculty member(s): _____

Date:_____   Time: _____   Duration:_____

Learning objective(s) of the session:

1. _____   2. _____

3. _____   4. _____

Teaching learning method(s):_____

REFLECTION

A. Please describe what happened during the session:

_____

_____

_____

_____

B. What did you learn from the session?

_____

_____

_____

_____

C. How will it help you become a better doctor in the future?

_____

_____

_____

_____

Skills Module: Session 11

Name of the session: _____

Name of the faculty member(s): _____

Date:_____   Time: _____   Duration:_____

Learning objective(s) of the session:

1. _____   2. _____

3. _____   4. _____

Teaching learning method(s):_____

REFLECTION

A. Please describe what happened during the session:

_____

_____

_____

_____

B. What did you learn from the session?

_____

_____

_____

_____

C. How will it help you become a better doctor in the future?

_____

_____

_____

_____

Skills Module: Session 12

Name of the session: _____

Name of the faculty member(s): _____

Date:_____   Time:_____   Duration:_____

Learning objective(s) of the session:

1. _____   2. _____

3. _____   4. _____

Teaching learning method(s):_____

REFLECTION

A. Please describe what happened during the session:

_____

_____

_____

_____

B. What did you learn from the session?

_____

_____

_____

_____

C. How will it help you become a better doctor in the future?

_____

_____

_____

_____

Skills Module: Session 13

Name of the session: _____

Name of the faculty member(s): _____

Date:_____   Time: _____   Duration:_____

Learning objective(s) of the session:

1. _____   2. _____

3. _____   4. _____

Teaching learning method(s): _____

REFLECTION

A. Please describe what happened during the session:

_____

_____

_____

_____

B. What did you learn from the session?

_____

_____

_____

_____

C. How will it help you become a better doctor in the future?

_____

_____

_____

Skills Module: Session 14

Name of the session: _____

Name of the faculty member(s): _____

Date:_____   Time: _____   Duration:_____

Learning objective(s) of the session:

1. _____   2. _____

3. _____   4. _____

Teaching learning method(s):_____

REFLECTION

A. Please describe what happened during the session:

_____

_____

_____

_____

B. What did you learn from the session?

_____

_____

_____

_____

C. How will it help you become a better doctor in the future?

_____

_____

_____

_____

Skills Module: Session 15

Name of the session: _____

Name of the faculty member(s): _____

Date:_____   Time: _____   Duration:_____

Learning objective(s) of the session:

1. _____   2. _____

3. _____   4. _____

Teaching learning method(s):_____

REFLECTION

A. Please describe what happened during the session:

_____

_____

_____

_____

B. What did you learn from the session?

_____

_____

_____

_____

C. How will it help you become a better doctor in the future?

_____

_____

_____

_____

Skills Module: Session 16

Name of the session: _____

Name of the faculty member(s): _____

Date: _____   Time: _____   Duration: _____

Learning objective(s) of the session:

1. _____   2. _____

3. _____   4. _____

Teaching learning method(s): _____

REFLECTION

A. Please describe what happened during the session:

_____

_____

_____

_____

B. What did you learn from the session?

_____

_____

_____

_____

C. How will it help you become a better doctor in the future?

_____

_____

_____

_____

Skills Module: Session 17

Name of the session: _____

Name of the faculty member(s): _____

Date:_____ Time: _____ Duration:_____

Learning objective(s) of the session:

1. _____ 2. _____

3. _____ 4. _____

Teaching learning method(s):_____

REFLECTION

A. Please describe what happened during the session:

_____

_____

_____

_____

B. What did you learn from the session?

_____

_____

_____

_____

C. How will it help you become a better doctor in the future?

_____

_____

_____

_____

Skills Module: Session 18

Name of the session: _____

Name of the faculty member(s): _____

Date:_____   Time:_____   Duration:_____

Learning objective(s) of the session:

1. _____   2. _____

3. _____   4. _____

Teaching learning method(s):_____

REFLECTION

A. Please describe what happened during the session:

_____

_____

_____

_____

B. What did you learn from the session?

_____

_____

_____

_____

C. How will it help you become a better doctor in the future?

_____

_____

_____

_____

Skills Module: Session 19

Name of the session: _____

Name of the faculty member(s): _____

Date: _____   Time: _____   Duration: _____

Learning objective(s) of the session:

1. _____   2. _____

3. _____   4. _____

Teaching learning method(s): _____

REFLECTION

A. Please describe what happened during the session:

_____

_____

_____

_____

B. What did you learn from the session?

_____

_____

_____

_____

C. How will it help you become a better doctor in the future?

_____

_____

_____

_____

Skills Module: Session 20

Name of the session: _____

Name of the faculty member(s): _____

Date: _____ Time: _____ Duration: _____

Learning objective(s) of the session:

1. _____ 2. _____

3. _____ 4. _____

Teaching learning method(s): _____

REFLECTION

A. Please describe what happened during the session:

_____

_____

_____

_____

B. What did you learn from the session?

_____

_____

_____

_____

C. How will it help you become a better doctor in the future?

_____

_____

_____

_____

Skills Module: Session 21

Name of the session: _____

Name of the faculty member(s): _____

Date:_____   Time: _____   Duration:_____

Learning objective(s) of the session:

1. _____   2. _____

3. _____   4. _____

Teaching learning method(s):_____

REFLECTION

A. Please describe what happened during the session:

_____

_____

_____

_____

B. What did you learn from the session?

_____

_____

_____

_____

C. How will it help you become a better doctor in the future?

_____

_____

_____

_____

Skills Module: Session 22

Name of the session: _____

Name of the faculty member(s): _____

Date: _____   Time: _____   Duration: _____

Learning objective(s) of the session:

1. _____   2. _____

3. _____   4. _____

Teaching learning method(s): _____

REFLECTION

A. Please describe what happened during the session:

_____

_____

_____

_____

B. What did you learn from the session?

_____

_____

_____

C. How will it help you become a better doctor in the future?

_____

_____

_____

_____

Skills Module: Session 23

Name of the session: _____

Name of the faculty member(s): _____

Date:_____   Time: _____   Duration:_____

Learning objective(s) of the session:

1. _____   2. _____

3. _____   4. _____

Teaching learning method(s):_____

REFLECTION

A. Please describe what happened during the session:

_____

_____

_____

_____

B. What did you learn from the session?

_____

_____

_____

_____

C. How will it help you become a better doctor in the future?

_____

_____

_____

_____

Skills Module: Session 24

Name of the session: _____

Name of the faculty member(s): _____

Date:_____   Time: _____   Duration:_____

Learning objective(s) of the session:

1. _____   2. _____

3. _____   4. _____

Teaching learning method(s):_____

REFLECTION

A. Please describe what happened during the session:

_____

_____

_____

_____

B. What did you learn from the session?

_____

_____

_____

_____

C. How will it help you become a better doctor in the future?

_____

_____

_____

_____

Skills Module: Session 25

Name of the session: _____

Name of the faculty member(s): _____

Date: _____ Time: _____ Duration: _____

Learning objective(s) of the session:

1. _____ 2. _____

3. _____ 4. _____

Teaching learning method(s): _____

REFLECTION

A. Please describe what happened during the session:

_____

_____

_____

_____

B. What did you learn from the session?

_____

_____

_____

_____

C. How will it help you become a better doctor in the future?

_____

_____

_____

Skills Module: Session 26

Name of the session: _____

Name of the faculty member(s): _____

Date:_____   Time:_____   Duration:_____

Learning objective(s) of the session:

1. _____   2. _____

3. _____   4. _____

Teaching learning method(s):_____

REFLECTION

A. Please describe what happened during the session:

_____

_____

_____

_____

B. What did you learn from the session?

_____

_____

_____

_____

C. How will it help you become a better doctor in the future?

_____

_____

_____

_____

Skills Module: Session 27

Name of the session: _____

Name of the faculty member(s): _____

Date:_____ Time: _____ Duration:_____

Learning objective(s) of the session:

1. _____ 2. _____

3. _____ 4. _____

Teaching learning method(s):_____

REFLECTION

A. Please describe what happened during the session:

_____

_____

_____

_____

B. What did you learn from the session?

_____

_____

_____

_____

C. How will it help you become a better doctor in the future?

_____

_____

_____

Skills Module: Session 28

Name of the session: _____

Name of the faculty member(s): _____

Date:_____   Time: _____   Duration:_____

Learning objective(s) of the session:

1. _____   2. _____

3. _____   4. _____

Teaching learning method(s):_____

REFLECTION

A. Please describe what happened during the session:

_____

_____

_____

_____

B. What did you learn from the session?

_____

_____

_____

_____

C. How will it help you become a better doctor in the future?

_____

_____

_____

_____

Skills Module: Session 29

Name of the session: _____

Name of the faculty member(s): _____

Date: _____   Time: _____   Duration: _____

Learning objective(s) of the session:

1. _____   2. _____

3. _____   4. _____

Teaching learning method(s): _____

REFLECTION

A. Please describe what happened during the session:

_____

_____

_____

_____

B. What did you learn from the session?

_____

_____

_____

_____

C. How will it help you become a better doctor in the future?

_____

_____

_____

_____

Skills Module: Session 30

Name of the session: _____

Name of the faculty member(s): _____

Date:_____   Time: _____   Duration:_____

Learning objective(s) of the session:

1. _____   2. _____

3. _____   4. _____

Teaching learning method(s):_____

REFLECTION

A. Please describe what happened during the session:

_____

_____

_____

_____

B. What did you learn from the session?

_____

_____

_____

_____

C. How will it help you become a better doctor in the future?

_____

_____

_____

_____

Skills Module: Session 31

Name of the session: _____

Name of the faculty member(s): _____

Date: _____ Time: _____ Duration: _____

Learning objective(s) of the session:

1. _____ 2. _____

3. _____ 4. _____

Teaching learning method(s): _____

REFLECTION

A. Please describe what happened during the session:

_____

_____

_____

_____

B. What did you learn from the session?

_____

_____

_____

_____

C. How will it help you become a better doctor in the future?

_____

_____

_____

Skills Module: Session 32

Name of the session: _____

Name of the faculty member(s): _____

Date: _____   Time: _____   Duration: _____

Learning objective(s) of the session:

1. _____   2. _____

3. _____   4. _____

Teaching learning method(s): _____

REFLECTION

A. Please describe what happened during the session:

_____

_____

_____

_____

B. What did you learn from the session?

_____

_____

_____

_____

C. How will it help you become a better doctor in the future?

_____

_____

_____

_____

Skills Module: Session 33

Name of the session: _____

Name of the faculty member(s): _____

Date: _____   Time: _____   Duration: _____

Learning objective(s) of the session:

1. _____   2. _____

3. _____   4. _____

Teaching learning method(s): _____

REFLECTION

A. Please describe what happened during the session:

_____

_____

_____

_____

B. What did you learn from the session?

_____

_____

_____

_____

C. How will it help you become a better doctor in the future?

_____

_____

_____

_____

Skills Module: Session 34

Name of the session: _____

Name of the faculty member(s): _____

Date:_____   Time: _____   Duration:_____

Learning objective(s) of the session:

1. _____   2. _____

3. _____   4. _____

Teaching learning method(s):_____

REFLECTION

A. Please describe what happened during the session:

_____

_____

_____

_____

B. What did you learn from the session?

_____

_____

_____

_____

C. How will it help you become a better doctor in the future?

_____

_____

_____

_____

Skills Module: Session 35

Name of the session: _____

Name of the faculty member(s): _____

Date:_____   Time:_____   Duration:_____

Learning objective(s) of the session:

1. _____   2. _____

3. _____   4. _____

Teaching learning method(s):_____

REFLECTION

A. Please describe what happened during the session:

_____

_____

_____

_____

B. What did you learn from the session?

_____

_____

_____

_____

C. How will it help you become a better doctor in the future?

_____

_____

_____

_____

Field Visits

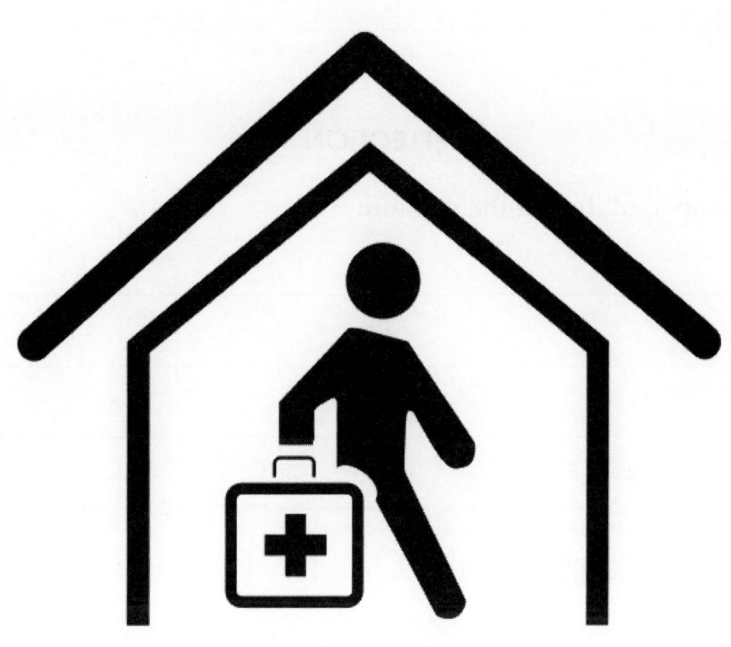

Field Visits: Session 1

Name of the session: _____

Name of the faculty member(s): _____

Date:_____   Time: _____   Duration:_____

Learning objective(s) of the session:

1. _____   2. _____

3. _____   4. _____

Teaching learning method(s):_____

REFLECTION

A. Please describe what happened during the session:

_____

_____

_____

_____

B. What did you learn from the session?

_____

_____

_____

_____

C. How will it help you become a better doctor in the future?

_____

_____

_____

Field Visits: Session 2

Name of the session: _____

Name of the faculty member(s): _____

Date:_____   Time: _____   Duration:_____

Learning objective(s) of the session:

1. _____   2. _____

3. _____   4. _____

Teaching learning method(s):_____

REFLECTION

A. Please describe what happened during the session:

_____

_____

_____

_____

B. What did you learn from the session?

_____

_____

_____

_____

C. How will it help you become a better doctor in the future?

_____

_____

_____

_____

Field Visits: Session 3

Name of the session: _____

Name of the faculty member(s): _____

Date:_____   Time: _____   Duration:_____

Learning objective(s) of the session:

1. _____   2. _____

3. _____   4. _____

Teaching learning method(s):_____

REFLECTION

A. Please describe what happened during the session:

_____

_____

_____

_____

B. What did you learn from the session?

_____

_____

_____

_____

C. How will it help you become a better doctor in the future?

_____

_____

_____

Field Visits: Session 4

Name of the session: _____

Name of the faculty member(s): _____

Date:_____   Time:_____   Duration:_____

Learning objective(s) of the session:

1. _____   2. _____

3. _____   4. _____

Teaching learning method(s):_____

REFLECTION

A. Please describe what happened during the session:

_____

_____

_____

_____

B. What did you learn from the session?

_____

_____

_____

_____

C. How will it help you become a better doctor in the future?

_____

_____

_____

_____

Field Visits: Session 5

Name of the session: _____

Name of the faculty member(s): _____

Date:_____   Time: _____   Duration:_____

Learning objective(s) of the session:

1. _____   2. _____

3. _____   4. _____

Teaching learning method(s):_____

REFLECTION

A. Please describe what happened during the session:

_____

_____

_____

_____

B. What did you learn from the session?

_____

_____

_____

_____

C. How will it help you become a better doctor in the future?

_____

_____

_____

_____

Field Visits: Session 6

Name of the session: _____

Name of the faculty member(s): _____

Date: _____   Time: _____   Duration: _____

Learning objective(s) of the session:

1. _____   2. _____

3. _____   4. _____

Teaching learning method(s): _____

REFLECTION

A. Please describe what happened during the session:

_____

_____

_____

_____

B. What did you learn from the session?

_____

_____

_____

_____

C. How will it help you become a better doctor in the future?

_____

_____

_____

_____

Field Visits: Session 7

Name of the session: _____

Name of the faculty member(s): _____

Date:_____   Time: _____   Duration:_____

Learning objective(s) of the session:

1. _____   2. _____

3. _____   4. _____

Teaching learning method(s):_____

REFLECTION

A. Please describe what happened during the session:

_____

_____

_____

_____

B. What did you learn from the session?

_____

_____

_____

_____

C. How will it help you become a better doctor in the future?

_____

_____

_____

_____

Field Visits: Session 8

Name of the session: _____

Name of the faculty member(s): _____

Date:_____   Time: _____   Duration:_____

Learning objective(s) of the session:

1. _____   2. _____

3. _____   4. _____

Teaching learning method(s):_____

REFLECTION

A. Please describe what happened during the session:

_____

_____

_____

_____

B. What did you learn from the session?

_____

_____

_____

_____

C. How will it help you become a better doctor in the future?

_____

_____

_____

_____

Professional Development

Total Time 40 Hours

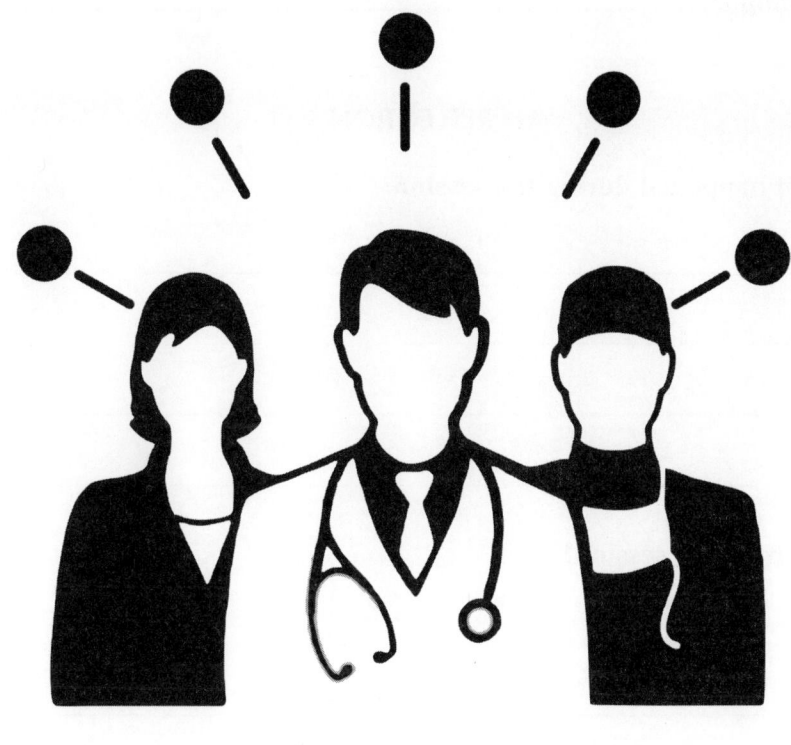

Professional Development: Session 1

Name of the session: _____

Name of the faculty member(s): _____

Date: _____   Time: _____   Duration: _____

Learning objective(s) of the session:

1. _____   2. _____

3. _____   4. _____

Teaching learning method(s): _____

REFLECTION

A. Please describe what happened during the session:

_____

_____

_____

_____

B. What did you learn from the session?

_____

_____

_____

_____

C. How will it help you become a better doctor in the future?

_____

_____

_____

_____

Professional Development: Session 2

Name of the session: _____

Name of the faculty member(s): _____

Date:_____   Time: _____   Duration:_____

Learning objective(s) of the session:

1. _____   2. _____

3. _____   4. _____

Teaching learning method(s):_____

REFLECTION

A. Please describe what happened during the session:

_____

_____

_____

_____

B. What did you learn from the session?

_____

_____

_____

_____

C. How will it help you become a better doctor in the future?

_____

_____

_____

_____

Professional Development: Session 3

Name of the session: _____

Name of the faculty member(s): _____

Date:_____   Time: _____   Duration:_____

Learning objective(s) of the session:

1. _____   2. _____

3. _____   4. _____

Teaching learning method(s):_____

REFLECTION

A. Please describe what happened during the session:

_____

_____

_____

_____

B. What did you learn from the session?

_____

_____

_____

_____

C. How will it help you become a better doctor in the future?

_____

_____

_____

_____

Professional Development: Session 4

Name of the session: _____

Name of the faculty member(s): _____

Date:_____   Time: _____   Duration:_____

Learning objective(s) of the session:

1. _____   2. _____

3. _____   4. _____

Teaching learning method(s):_____

REFLECTION

A. Please describe what happened during the session:

_____

_____

_____

_____

B. What did you learn from the session?

_____

_____

_____

_____

C. How will it help you become a better doctor in the future?

_____

_____

_____

_____

Professional Development: Session 5

Name of the session: _____

Name of the faculty member(s): _____

Date: _____   Time: _____   Duration: _____

Learning objective(s) of the session:

1. _____   2. _____

3. _____   4. _____

Teaching learning method(s): _____

REFLECTION

A. Please describe what happened during the session:

_____

_____

_____

_____

B. What did you learn from the session?

_____

_____

_____

C. How will it help you become a better doctor in the future?

_____

_____

_____

_____

Professional Development: Session 6

Name of the session: _____

Name of the faculty member(s): _____

Date:_____   Time: _____   Duration:_____

Learning objective(s) of the session:

1. _____   2. _____

3. _____   4. _____

Teaching learning method(s):_____

REFLECTION

A. Please describe what happened during the session:

_____

_____

_____

_____

B. What did you learn from the session?

_____

_____

_____

_____

C. How will it help you become a better doctor in the future?

_____

_____

_____

_____

Professional Development: Session 7

Name of the session: _____

Name of the faculty member(s): _____

Date:_____   Time: _____   Duration:_____

Learning objective(s) of the session:

1. _____   2. _____

3. _____   4. _____

Teaching learning method(s):_____

REFLECTION

A. Please describe what happened during the session:

_____

_____

_____

_____

B. What did you learn from the session?

_____

_____

_____

_____

C. How will it help you become a better doctor in the future?

_____

_____

_____

_____

Professional Development: Session 8

Name of the session: _____

Name of the faculty member(s): _____

Date:_____   Time: _____   Duration:_____

Learning objective(s) of the session:

1. _____   2. _____

3. _____   4. _____

Teaching learning method(s):_____

REFLECTION

A. Please describe what happened during the session:

_____

_____

_____

_____

B. What did you learn from the session?

_____

_____

_____

_____

C. How will it help you become a better doctor in the future?

_____

_____

_____

_____

Professional Development: Session 9

Name of the session: _____

Name of the faculty member(s): _____

Date:_____   Time:_____   Duration:_____

Learning objective(s) of the session:

1. _____   2. _____

3. _____   4. _____

Teaching learning method(s):_____

REFLECTION

A. Please describe what happened during the session:

_____

_____

_____

_____

B. What did you learn from the session?

_____

_____

_____

_____

C. How will it help you become a better doctor in the future?

_____

_____

_____

_____

Professional Development: Session 10

Name of the session: _____

Name of the faculty member(s): _____

Date: _____ Time: _____ Duration: _____

Learning objective(s) of the session:

1. _____ 2. _____

3. _____ 4. _____

Teaching learning method(s): _____

REFLECTION

A. Please describe what happened during the session:

_____

_____

_____

_____

B. What did you learn from the session?

_____

_____

_____

_____

C. How will it help you become a better doctor in the future?

_____

_____

_____

_____

Professional Development: Session 11

Name of the session: _____

Name of the faculty member(s): _____

Date: _____   Time: _____   Duration: _____

Learning objective(s) of the session:

1. _____   2. _____

3. _____   4. _____

Teaching learning method(s): _____

REFLECTION

A. Please describe what happened during the session:

_____

_____

_____

_____

B. What did you learn from the session?

_____

_____

_____

_____

C. How will it help you become a better doctor in the future?

_____

_____

_____

_____

Professional Development: Session 12

Name of the session: _____

Name of the faculty member(s): _____

Date:_____ Time:_____ Duration:_____

Learning objective(s) of the session:

1. _____ 2. _____

3. _____ 4. _____

Teaching learning method(s):_____

REFLECTION

A. Please describe what happened during the session:

_____

_____

_____

_____

B. What did you learn from the session?

_____

_____

_____

_____

C. How will it help you become a better doctor in the future?

_____

_____

_____

_____

Professional Development: Session 13

Name of the session: _____

Name of the faculty member(s): _____

Date: _____   Time: _____   Duration: _____

Learning objective(s) of the session:

1. _____   2. _____

3. _____   4. _____

Teaching learning method(s): _____

REFLECTION

A. Please describe what happened during the session:

_____

_____

_____

_____

B. What did you learn from the session?

_____

_____

_____

_____

C. How will it help you become a better doctor in the future?

_____

_____

_____

_____

Professional Development: Session 14

Name of the session: _____

Name of the faculty member(s): _____

Date: _____ Time: _____ Duration: _____

Learning objective(s) of the session:

1. _____ 2. _____

3. _____ 4. _____

Teaching learning method(s): _____

REFLECTION

A. Please describe what happened during the session:

_____

_____

_____

_____

B. What did you learn from the session?

_____

_____

_____

_____

C. How will it help you become a better doctor in the future?

_____

_____

_____

_____

Professional Development: Session 15

Name of the session: _____

Name of the faculty member(s): _____

Date:_____   Time: _____   Duration:_____

Learning objective(s) of the session:

1. _____   2. _____

3. _____   4. _____

Teaching learning method(s):_____

REFLECTION

A. Please describe what happened during the session:

_____

_____

_____

_____

B. What did you learn from the session?

_____

_____

_____

C. How will it help you become a better doctor in the future?

_____

_____

_____

Professional Development: Session 16

Name of the session: _____

Name of the faculty member(s): _____

Date:_____ Time: _____ Duration:_____

Learning objective(s) of the session:

1. _____   2. _____

3. _____   4. _____

Teaching learning method(s):_____

REFLECTION

A. Please describe what happened during the session:

_____

_____

_____

_____

B. What did you learn from the session?

_____

_____

_____

_____

C. How will it help you become a better doctor in the future?

_____

_____

_____

_____

Professional Development: Session 17

Name of the session: _____

Name of the faculty member(s): _____

Date:_____   Time:_____   Duration:_____

Learning objective(s) of the session:

1. _____   2. _____

3. _____   4. _____

Teaching learning method(s):_____

REFLECTION

A. Please describe what happened during the session:

_____

_____

_____

_____

B. What did you learn from the session?

_____

_____

_____

_____

C. How will it help you become a better doctor in the future?

_____

_____

_____

_____

Professional Development: Session 18

Name of the session: _____

Name of the faculty member(s): _____

Date: _____   Time: _____   Duration: _____

Learning objective(s) of the session:

1. _____   2. _____

3. _____   4. _____

Teaching learning method(s): _____

REFLECTION

A. Please describe what happened during the session:

_____

_____

_____

_____

B. What did you learn from the session?

_____

_____

_____

_____

C. How will it help you become a better doctor in the future?

_____

_____

_____

_____

Professional Development: Session 19

Name of the session: _____

Name of the faculty member(s): _____

Date:_____   Time:_____   Duration:_____

Learning objective(s) of the session:

1. _____   2. _____

3. _____   4. _____

Teaching learning method(s): _____

REFLECTION

A. Please describe what happened during the session:

_____

_____

_____

_____

B. What did you learn from the session?

_____

_____

_____

_____

C. How will it help you become a better doctor in the future?

_____

_____

_____

Professional Development: Session 20

Name of the session: _____

Name of the faculty member(s): _____

Date:_____   Time:_____   Duration:_____

Learning objective(s) of the session:

1. _____   2. _____

3. _____   4. _____

Teaching learning method(s):_____

REFLECTION

A. Please describe what happened during the session:

_____

_____

_____

_____

B. What did you learn from the session?

_____

_____

_____

C. How will it help you become a better doctor in the future?

_____

_____

_____

_____

Professional Development: Session 21

Name of the session: _____

Name of the faculty member(s): _____

Date:_____ Time: _____ Duration:_____

Learning objective(s) of the session:

1. _____ 2. _____

3. _____ 4. _____

Teaching learning method(s):_____

REFLECTION

A. Please describe what happened during the session:

_____

_____

_____

_____

B. What did you learn from the session?

_____

_____

_____

C. How will it help you become a better doctor in the future?

_____

_____

_____

_____

Professional Development: Session 22

Name of the session: _____

Name of the faculty member(s): _____

Date:_____   Time: _____   Duration:_____

Learning objective(s) of the session:

1. _____   2. _____

3. _____   4. _____

Teaching learning method(s):_____

REFLECTION

A. Please describe what happened during the session:

_____

_____

_____

_____

B. What did you learn from the session?

_____

_____

_____

_____

C. How will it help you become a better doctor in the future?

_____

_____

_____

_____

Professional Development: Session 23

Name of the session: _____

Name of the faculty member(s): _____

Date:_____   Time: _____   Duration:_____

Learning objective(s) of the session:

1. _____   2. _____

3. _____   4. _____

Teaching learning method(s):_____

REFLECTION

A. Please describe what happened during the session:

_____

_____

_____

_____

B. What did you learn from the session?

_____

_____

_____

_____

C. How will it help you become a better doctor in the future?

_____

_____

_____

_____

Professional Development: Session 24

Name of the session: _____

Name of the faculty member(s): _____

Date:_____   Time:_____   Duration:_____

Learning objective(s) of the session:

1. _____   2. _____

3. _____   4. _____

Teaching learning method(s):_____

REFLECTION

A. Please describe what happened during the session:

_____

_____

_____

_____

B. What did you learn from the session?

_____

_____

_____

_____

C. How will it help you become a better doctor in the future?

_____

_____

_____

_____

Professional Development: Session 25

Name of the session: _____

Name of the faculty member(s): _____

Date:_____   Time: _____   Duration:_____

Learning objective(s) of the session:

1. _____   2. _____

3. _____   4. _____

Teaching learning method(s):_____

REFLECTION

A. Please describe what happened during the session:

_____

_____

_____

_____

B. What did you learn from the session?

_____

_____

_____

_____

C. How will it help you become a better doctor in the future?

_____

_____

_____

_____

Professional Development: Session 26

Name of the session: _____

Name of the faculty member(s): _____

Date:_____   Time: _____   Duration:_____

Learning objective(s) of the session:

1. _____   2. _____

3. _____   4. _____

Teaching learning method(s): _____

REFLECTION

A. Please describe what happened during the session:

_____

_____

_____

_____

B. What did you learn from the session?

_____

_____

_____

_____

C. How will it help you become a better doctor in the future?

_____

_____

_____

_____

Professional Development: Session 27

Name of the session: _____

Name of the faculty member(s): _____

Date:_____ **Time:** _____ **Duration:**_____

Learning objective(s) of the session:

1. _____ 2. _____

3. _____ 4. _____

Teaching learning method(s):_____

REFLECTION

A. Please describe what happened during the session:

_____

_____

_____

_____

B. What did you learn from the session?

_____

_____

_____

_____

C. How will it help you become a better doctor in the future?

_____

_____

_____

_____

Professional Development: Session 28

Name of the session: _____

Name of the faculty member(s): _____

Date: _____   Time: _____   Duration: _____

Learning objective(s) of the session:

1. _____   2. _____

3. _____   4. _____

Teaching learning method(s): _____

REFLECTION

A. Please describe what happened during the session:

_____

_____

_____

_____

B. What did you learn from the session?

_____

_____

_____

_____

C. How will it help you become a better doctor in the future?

_____

_____

_____

_____

Professional Development: Session 29

Name of the session: _____

Name of the faculty member(s): _____

Date:_____   Time: _____   Duration:_____

Learning objective(s) of the session:

1. _____   2. _____

3. _____   4. _____

Teaching learning method(s):_____

REFLECTION

A. Please describe what happened during the session:

_____

_____

_____

_____

B. What did you learn from the session?

_____

_____

_____

_____

C. How will it help you become a better doctor in the future?

_____

_____

_____

_____

Professional Development: Session 30

Name of the session: _____

Name of the faculty member(s): _____

Date: _____   Time: _____   Duration: _____

Learning objective(s) of the session:

1. _____   2. _____

3. _____   4. _____

Teaching learning method(s): _____

REFLECTION

A. Please describe what happened during the session:

_____

_____

_____

_____

B. What did you learn from the session?

_____

_____

_____

_____

C. How will it help you become a better doctor in the future?

_____

_____

_____

_____

Professional Development: Session 31

Name of the session: _____

Name of the faculty member(s): _____

Date:_____   Time: _____   Duration:_____

Learning objective(s) of the session:

1. _____   2. _____

3. _____   4. _____

Teaching learning method(s):_____

REFLECTION

A. Please describe what happened during the session:

_____

_____

_____

_____

B. What did you learn from the session?

_____

_____

_____

_____

C. How will it help you become a better doctor in the future?

_____

_____

_____

_____

Professional Development: Session 32

Name of the session: _____

Name of the faculty member(s): _____

Date: _____   Time: _____   Duration: _____

Learning objective(s) of the session:

1. _____   2. _____

3. _____   4. _____

Teaching learning method(s): _____

REFLECTION

A. Please describe what happened during the session:

_____

_____

_____

_____

B. What did you learn from the session?

_____

_____

_____

_____

C. How will it help you become a better doctor in the future?

_____

_____

_____

_____

Professional Development: Session 33

Name of the session: _____

Name of the faculty member(s): _____

Date:_____ Time: _____ Duration:_____

Learning objective(s) of the session:

1. _____ 2. _____

3. _____ 4. _____

Teaching learning method(s):_____

REFLECTION

A. Please describe what happened during the session:

_____

_____

_____

_____

B. What did you learn from the session?

_____

_____

_____

_____

C. How will it help you become a better doctor in the future?

_____

_____

_____

_____

Professional Development: Session 34

Name of the session: _____

Name of the faculty member(s): _____

Date: _____ Time: _____ Duration: _____

Learning objective(s) of the session:

1. _____ 2. _____

3. _____ 4. _____

Teaching learning method(s): _____

REFLECTION

A. Please describe what happened during the session:

_____

_____

_____

_____

B. What did you learn from the session?

_____

_____

_____

_____

C. How will it help you become a better doctor in the future?

_____

_____

_____

_____

Professional Development: Session 35

Name of the session: _____

Name of the faculty member(s): _____

Date:_____   Time:_____   Duration:_____

Learning objective(s) of the session:

1. _____   2. _____

3. _____   4. _____

Teaching learning method(s):_____

REFLECTION

A. Please describe what happened during the session:

_____

_____

_____

_____

B. What did you learn from the session?

_____

_____

_____

_____

C. How will it help you become a better doctor in the future?

_____

_____

_____

_____

Professional Development: Session 36

Name of the session: _____

Name of the faculty member(s): _____

Date:_____   Time: _____   Duration:_____

Learning objective(s) of the session:

1. _____   2. _____

3. _____   4. _____

Teaching learning method(s):_____

REFLECTION

A. Please describe what happened during the session:

_____

_____

_____

_____

B. What did you learn from the session?

_____

_____

_____

_____

C. How will it help you become a better doctor in the future?

_____

_____

_____

_____

Professional Development: Session 37

Name of the session: _____

Name of the faculty member(s): _____

Date:_____   Time: _____   Duration:_____

Learning objective(s) of the session:

1. _____   2. _____

3. _____   4. _____

Teaching learning method(s):_____

REFLECTION

A. Please describe what happened during the session:

_____

_____

_____

_____

B. What did you learn from the session?

_____

_____

_____

_____

C. How will it help you become a better doctor in the future?

_____

_____

_____

_____

Professional Development: Session 38

Name of the session: _____

Name of the faculty member(s): _____

Date:_____ Time: _____ Duration:_____

Learning objective(s) of the session:

1. _____ 2. _____

3. _____ 4. _____

Teaching learning method(s):_____

REFLECTION

A. Please describe what happened during the session:

_____

_____

_____

_____

B. What did you learn from the session?

_____

_____

_____

_____

C. How will it help you become a better doctor in the future?

_____

_____

_____

_____

Professional Development: Session 39

Name of the session: _____

Name of the faculty member(s): _____

Date: _____   Time: _____   Duration: _____

Learning objective(s) of the session:

1. _____   2. _____

3. _____   4. _____

Teaching learning method(s): _____

REFLECTION

A. Please describe what happened during the session:

_____

_____

_____

_____

B. What did you learn from the session?

_____

_____

_____

_____

C. How will it help you become a better doctor in the future?

_____

_____

_____

_____

Professional Development: Session 40

Name of the session: _____

Name of the faculty member(s): _____

Date:_____   Time: _____   Duration:_____

Learning objective(s) of the session:

1. _____   2. _____

3. _____   4. _____

Teaching learning method(s):_____

REFLECTION

A. Please describe what happened during the session:

_____

_____

_____

_____

B. What did you learn from the session?

_____

_____

_____

_____

C. How will it help you become a better doctor in the future?

_____

_____

_____

_____

Language and Computer Skills

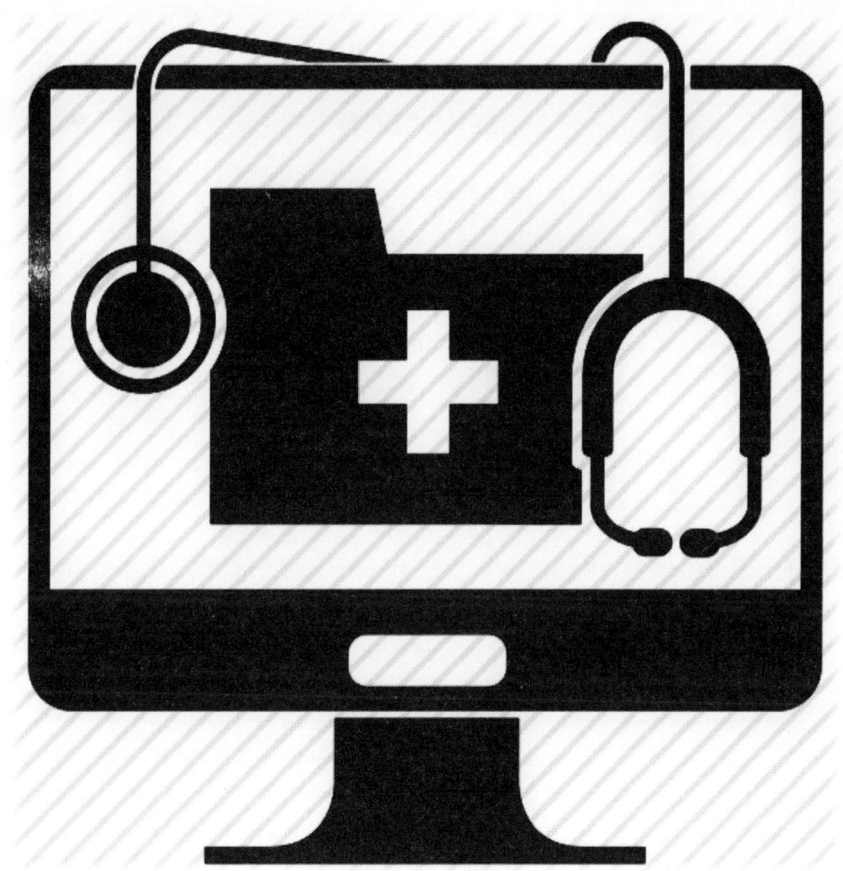

Language and Computer Skills: Session 1

Name of the session: _____

Name of the faculty member(s): _____

Date:_____ Time: _____ Duration:_____

Learning objective(s) of the session:

1. _____ 2. _____

3. _____ 4. _____

Teaching learning method(s):_____

REFLECTION

A. Please describe what happened during the session:

_____

_____

_____

_____

B. What did you learn from the session?

_____

_____

_____

_____

C. How will it help you become a better doctor in the future?

_____

_____

_____

_____

Language and Computer Skills: Session 2

Name of the session: _____

Name of the faculty member(s): _____

Date:_____   Time: _____   Duration:_____

Learning objective(s) of the session:

1. _____   2. _____

3. _____   4. _____

Teaching learning method(s):_____

REFLECTION

A. Please describe what happened during the session:

_____

_____

_____

_____

B. What did you learn from the session?

_____

_____

_____

_____

C. How will it help you become a better doctor in the future?

_____

_____

_____

_____

Language and Computer Skills: Session 3

Name of the session: _____

Name of the faculty member(s): _____

Date:_____   Time: _____   Duration:_____

Learning objective(s) of the session:

1. _____   2. _____

3. _____   4. _____

Teaching learning method(s):_____

REFLECTION

A. Please describe what happened during the session:

_____

_____

_____

_____

B. What did you learn from the session?

_____

_____

_____

_____

C. How will it help you become a better doctor in the future?

_____

_____

_____

_____

Language and Computer Skills: Session 4

Name of the session: _____

Name of the faculty member(s): _____

Date:_____   Time: _____   Duration:_____

Learning objective(s) of the session:

1. _____   2. _____

3. _____   4. _____

Teaching learning method(s):_____

REFLECTION

A. Please describe what happened during the session:

_____

_____

_____

_____

B. What did you learn from the session?

_____

_____

_____

_____

C. How will it help you become a better doctor in the future?

_____

_____

_____

_____

Language and Computer Skills: Session 5

Name of the session: _____

Name of the faculty member(s): _____

Date:_____   Time: _____   Duration:_____

Learning objective(s) of the session:

1. _____   2. _____

3. _____   4. _____

Teaching learning method(s):_____

REFLECTION

A. Please describe what happened during the session:

_____

_____

_____

_____

B. What did you learn from the session?

_____

_____

_____

_____

C. How will it help you become a better doctor in the future?

_____

_____

_____

_____

Language and Computer Skills: Session 6

Name of the session: _____

Name of the faculty member(s): _____

Date: _____   Time: _____   Duration: _____

Learning objective(s) of the session:

1. _____   2. _____

3. _____   4. _____

Teaching learning method(s): _____

REFLECTION

A. Please describe what happened during the session:

_____

_____

_____

_____

B. What did you learn from the session?

_____

_____

_____

_____

C. How will it help you become a better doctor in the future?

_____

_____

_____

_____

Language and Computer Skills: Session 7

Name of the session: _____

Name of the faculty member(s): _____

Date: _____   Time: _____   Duration: _____

Learning objective(s) of the session:

1. _____   2. _____

3. _____   4. _____

Teaching learning method(s): _____

REFLECTION

A. Please describe what happened during the session:

_____

_____

_____

_____

B. What did you learn from the session?

_____

_____

_____

_____

C. How will it help you become a better doctor in the future?

_____

_____

_____

_____

Language and Computer Skills: Session 8

Name of the session: _____

Name of the faculty member(s): _____

Date:_____   Time: _____   Duration:_____

Learning objective(s) of the session:

1. _____   2. _____

3. _____   4. _____

Teaching learning method(s): _____

REFLECTION

A. Please describe what happened during the session:

_____

_____

_____

_____

B. What did you learn from the session?

_____

_____

_____

_____

C. How will it help you become a better doctor in the future?

_____

_____

_____

_____

Language and Computer Skills: Session 9

Name of the session: _____

Name of the faculty member(s): _____

Date:_____   Time: _____   Duration:_____

Learning objective(s) of the session:

1. _____   2. _____

3. _____   4. _____

Teaching learning method(s):_____

REFLECTION

A. Please describe what happened during the session:

_____

_____

_____

_____

B. What did you learn from the session?

_____

_____

_____

C. How will it help you become a better doctor in the future?

_____

_____

_____

_____

Language and Computer Skills: Session 10

Name of the session: _____

Name of the faculty member(s): _____

Date:_____   Time: _____   Duration:_____

Learning objective(s) of the session:

1. _____   2. _____

3. _____   4. _____

Teaching learning method(s):_____

REFLECTION

A. Please describe what happened during the session:

_____

_____

_____

_____

B. What did you learn from the session?

_____

_____

_____

_____

C. How will it help you become a better doctor in the future?

_____

_____

_____

_____

Language and Computer Skills: Session 11

Name of the session: _____

Name of the faculty member(s): _____

Date:_____   Time: _____   Duration:_____

Learning objective(s) of the session:

1. _____   2. _____

3. _____   4. _____

Teaching learning method(s):_____

REFLECTION

A. Please describe what happened during the session:

_____

_____

_____

_____

B. What did you learn from the session?

_____

_____

_____

_____

C. How will it help you become a better doctor in the future?

_____

_____

_____

_____

Language and Computer Skills: Session 12

Name of the session: _____

Name of the faculty member(s): _____

Date:_____   Time: _____   Duration:_____

Learning objective(s) of the session:

1. _____   2. _____

3. _____   4. _____

Teaching learning method(s):_____

REFLECTION

A. Please describe what happened during the session:

_____

_____

_____

_____

B. What did you learn from the session?

_____

_____

_____

_____

C. How will it help you become a better doctor in the future?

_____

_____

_____

_____

Language and Computer Skills: Session 13

Name of the session: _____

Name of the faculty member(s): _____

Date:_____ Time:_____ Duration:_____

Learning objective(s) of the session:

1. _____ 2. _____

3. _____ 4. _____

Teaching learning method(s):_____

REFLECTION

A. Please describe what happened during the session:

_____

_____

_____

_____

B. What did you learn from the session?

_____

_____

_____

_____

C. How will it help you become a better doctor in the future?

_____

_____

_____

_____

Language and Computer Skills: Session 14

Name of the session: _____

Name of the faculty member(s): _____

Date: _____   Time: _____   Duration: _____

Learning objective(s) of the session:

1. _____   2. _____

3. _____   4. _____

Teaching learning method(s): _____

REFLECTION

A. Please describe what happened during the session:

_____

_____

_____

_____

B. What did you learn from the session?

_____

_____

_____

_____

C. How will it help you become a better doctor in the future?

_____

_____

_____

_____

Language and Computer Skills: Session 15

Name of the session: _____

Name of the faculty member(s): _____

Date: _____ Time: _____ Duration: _____

Learning objective(s) of the session:

1. _____ 2. _____

3. _____ 4. _____

Teaching learning method(s): _____

REFLECTION

A. Please describe what happened during the session:

_____

_____

_____

_____

B. What did you learn from the session?

_____

_____

_____

_____

C. How will it help you become a better doctor in the future?

_____

_____

_____

_____

Language and Computer Skills: Session 16

Name of the session: _____

Name of the faculty member(s): _____

Date:_____   Time: _____   Duration:_____

Learning objective(s) of the session:

1. _____   2. _____

3. _____   4. _____

Teaching learning method(s):_____

REFLECTION

A. Please describe what happened during the session:

_____

_____

_____

_____

B. What did you learn from the session?

_____

_____

_____

_____

C. How will it help you become a better doctor in the future?

_____

_____

_____

_____

Language and Computer Skills: Session 17

Name of the session: _____

Name of the faculty member(s): _____

Date: _____   Time: _____   Duration: _____

Learning objective(s) of the session:

1. _____   2. _____

3. _____   4. _____

Teaching learning method(s): _____

REFLECTION

A. Please describe what happened during the session:

_____

_____

_____

_____

B. What did you learn from the session?

_____

_____

_____

_____

C. How will it help you become a better doctor in the future?

_____

_____

_____

_____

Language and Computer Skills: Session 18

Name of the session: _____

Name of the faculty member(s): _____

Date:_____   Time: _____   Duration:_____

Learning objective(s) of the session:

1. _____   2. _____

3. _____   4. _____

Teaching learning method(s):_____

REFLECTION

A. Please describe what happened during the session:

_____

_____

_____

_____

B. What did you learn from the session?

_____

_____

_____

_____

C. How will it help you become a better doctor in the future?

_____

_____

_____

_____

Language and Computer Skills: Session 19

Name of the session: _____

Name of the faculty member(s): _____

Date:_____   Time: _____   Duration:_____

Learning objective(s) of the session:

1. _____   2. _____

3. _____   4. _____

Teaching learning method(s):_____

REFLECTION

A. Please describe what happened during the session:

_____

_____

_____

_____

B. What did you learn from the session?

_____

_____

_____

_____

C. How will it help you become a better doctor in the future?

_____

_____

_____

_____

Language and Computer Skills: Session 20

Name of the session: _____

Name of the faculty member(s): _____

Date:_____   Time: _____   Duration:_____

Learning objective(s) of the session:

1. _____   2. _____

3. _____   4. _____

Teaching learning method(s):_____

REFLECTION

A. Please describe what happened during the session:

_____

_____

_____

_____

B. What did you learn from the session?

_____

_____

_____

_____

C. How will it help you become a better doctor in the future?

_____

_____

_____

Language and Computer Skills: Session 21

Name of the session: _____

Name of the faculty member(s): _____

Date: _____ Time: _____ Duration: _____

Learning objective(s) of the session:

1. _____ 2. _____

3. _____ 4. _____

Teaching learning method(s): _____

REFLECTION

A. Please describe what happened during the session:

_____

_____

_____

_____

B. What did you learn from the session?

_____

_____

_____

C. How will it help you become a better doctor in the future?

_____

_____

_____

_____

Language and Computer Skills: Session 22

Name of the session: _____

Name of the faculty member(s): _____

Date:_____   Time: _____   Duration:_____

Learning objective(s) of the session:

1. _____   2. _____

3. _____   4. _____

Teaching learning method(s):_____

REFLECTION

A. Please describe what happened during the session:

_____

_____

_____

_____

B. What did you learn from the session?

_____

_____

_____

_____

C. How will it help you become a better doctor in the future?

_____

_____

_____

_____

Language and Computer Skills: Session 23

Name of the session: _____

Name of the faculty member(s): _____

Date: _____   Time: _____   Duration: _____

Learning objective(s) of the session:

1. _____   2. _____

3. _____   4. _____

Teaching learning method(s): _____

REFLECTION

A. Please describe what happened during the session:

_____

_____

_____

_____

B. What did you learn from the session?

_____

_____

_____

_____

C. How will it help you become a better doctor in the future?

_____

_____

_____

_____

Language and Computer Skills: Session 24

Name of the session: _____

Name of the faculty member(s): _____

Date:_____   Time: _____   Duration:_____

Learning objective(s) of the session:

1. _____   2. _____

3. _____   4. _____

Teaching learning method(s):_____

REFLECTION

A. Please describe what happened during the session:

_____

_____

_____

_____

B. What did you learn from the session?

_____

_____

_____

_____

C. How will it help you become a better doctor in the future?

_____

_____

_____

_____

Language and Computer Skills: Session 25

Name of the session: _____

Name of the faculty member(s): _____

Date:_____   Time: _____   Duration:_____

Learning objective(s) of the session:

1. _____   2. _____

3. _____   4. _____

Teaching learning method(s):_____

REFLECTION

A. Please describe what happened during the session:

_____

_____

_____

_____

B. What did you learn from the session?

_____

_____

_____

_____

C. How will it help you become a better doctor in the future?

_____

_____

_____

_____

Language and Computer Skills: Session 26

Name of the session: _____

Name of the faculty member(s): _____

Date:_____   Time: _____   Duration:_____

Learning objective(s) of the session:

1. _____   2. _____

3. _____   4. _____

Teaching learning method(s):_____

REFLECTION

A. Please describe what happened during the session:

_____

_____

_____

_____

B. What did you learn from the session?

_____

_____

_____

_____

C. How will it help you become a better doctor in the future?

_____

_____

_____

_____

Language and Computer Skills: Session 27

Name of the session: _____

Name of the faculty member(s): _____

Date: _____ Time: _____ Duration: _____

Learning objective(s) of the session:

1. _____ 2. _____

3. _____ 4. _____

Teaching learning method(s): _____

REFLECTION

A. Please describe what happened during the session:

_____

_____

_____

_____

B. What did you learn from the session?

_____

_____

_____

_____

C. How will it help you become a better doctor in the future?

_____

_____

_____

_____

Language and Computer Skills: Session 28

Name of the session: _____

Name of the faculty member(s): _____

Date:_____   Time: _____   Duration:_____

Learning objective(s) of the session:

1. _____   2. _____

3. _____   4. _____

Teaching learning method(s):_____

REFLECTION

A. Please describe what happened during the session:

_____

_____

_____

_____

B. What did you learn from the session?

_____

_____

_____

_____

C. How will it help you become a better doctor in the future?

_____

_____

_____

_____

Language and Computer Skills: Session 29

Name of the session: _____

Name of the faculty member(s): _____

Date:_____   Time:_____   Duration:_____

Learning objective(s) of the session:

1. _____   2. _____

3. _____   4. _____

Teaching learning method(s):_____

REFLECTION

A. Please describe what happened during the session:

_____

_____

_____

_____

B. What did you learn from the session?

_____

_____

_____

_____

C. How will it help you become a better doctor in the future?

_____

_____

_____

_____

Language and Computer Skills: Session 30

Name of the session: _____

Name of the faculty member(s): _____

Date:_____   Time: _____   Duration:_____

Learning objective(s) of the session:

1. _____   2. _____

3. _____   4. _____

Teaching learning method(s):_____

REFLECTION

A. Please describe what happened during the session:

_____

_____

_____

_____

B. What did you learn from the session?

_____

_____

_____

_____

C. How will it help you become a better doctor in the future?

_____

_____

_____

_____

Language and Computer Skills: Session 31

Name of the session: _____

Name of the faculty member(s): _____

Date:_____   Time: _____   Duration:_____

Learning objective(s) of the session:

1. _____   2. _____

3. _____   4. _____

Teaching learning method(s):_____

REFLECTION

A. Please describe what happened during the session:

_____

_____

_____

_____

B. What did you learn from the session?

_____

_____

_____

_____

C. How will it help you become a better doctor in the future?

_____

_____

_____

_____

Language and Computer Skills: Session 32

Name of the session: _____

Name of the faculty member(s): _____

Date:_____   Time:_____   Duration:_____

Learning objective(s) of the session:

1. _____   2. _____

3. _____   4. _____

Teaching learning method(s):_____

REFLECTION

A. Please describe what happened during the session:

_____

_____

_____

_____

B. What did you learn from the session?

_____

_____

_____

_____

C. How will it help you become a better doctor in the future?

_____

_____

_____

_____

Language and Computer Skills: Session 33

Name of the session: _____

Name of the faculty member(s): _____

Date:_____   Time:_____   Duration:_____

Learning objective(s) of the session:

1. _____   2. _____

3. _____   4. _____

Teaching learning method(s):_____

REFLECTION

A. Please describe what happened during the session:

_____

_____

_____

_____

B. What did you learn from the session?

_____

_____

_____

_____

C. How will it help you become a better doctor in the future?

_____

_____

_____

Language and Computer Skills: Session 34

Name of the session: _____

Name of the faculty member(s): _____

Date:_____   Time: _____   Duration:_____

Learning objective(s) of the session:

1. _____   2. _____

3. _____   4. _____

Teaching learning method(s):_____

REFLECTION

A. Please describe what happened during the session:

_____

_____

_____

_____

B. What did you learn from the session?

_____

_____

_____

C. How will it help you become a better doctor in the future?

_____

_____

_____

_____

Language and Computer Skills: Session 35

Name of the session: _____

Name of the faculty member(s): _____

Date:_____   Time: _____   Duration:_____

Learning objective(s) of the session:

1. _____   2. _____

3. _____   4. _____

Teaching learning method(s):_____

REFLECTION

A. Please describe what happened during the session:

_____

_____

_____

_____

B. What did you learn from the session?

_____

_____

_____

_____

C. How will it help you become a better doctor in the future?

_____

_____

_____

_____

Language and Computer Skills: Session 36

Name of the session: _____

Name of the faculty member(s): _____

Date:_____ Time: _____ Duration:_____

Learning objective(s) of the session:

1. _____ 2. _____

3. _____ 4. _____

Teaching learning method(s):_____

REFLECTION

A. Please describe what happened during the session:

_____

_____

_____

_____

B. What did you learn from the session?

_____

_____

_____

_____

C. How will it help you become a better doctor in the future?

_____

_____

_____

_____

Language and Computer Skills: Session 37

Name of the session: _____

Name of the faculty member(s): _____

Date:_____   Time:_____   Duration:_____

Learning objective(s) of the session:

1. _____   2. _____

3. _____   4. _____

Teaching learning method(s):_____

REFLECTION

A. Please describe what happened during the session:

_____

_____

_____

_____

B. What did you learn from the session?

_____

_____

_____

_____

C. How will it help you become a better doctor in the future?

_____

_____

_____

_____

Language and Computer Skills: Session 38

Name of the session: _____

Name of the faculty member(s): _____

Date: _____   Time: _____   Duration: _____

Learning objective(s) of the session:

1. _____   2. _____

3. _____   4. _____

Teaching learning method(s): _____

REFLECTION

A. Please describe what happened during the session:

_____

_____

_____

_____

B. What did you learn from the session?

_____

_____

_____

_____

C. How will it help you become a better doctor in the future?

_____

_____

_____

_____

Language and Computer Skills: Session 39

Name of the session: _____

Name of the faculty member(s): _____

Date:_____   Time: _____   Duration:_____

Learning objective(s) of the session:

1. _____   2. _____

3. _____   4. _____

Teaching learning method(s):_____

REFLECTION

A. Please describe what happened during the session:

_____

_____

_____

_____

B. What did you learn from the session?

_____

_____

_____

_____

C. How will it help you become a better doctor in the future?

_____

_____

_____

_____

Language and Computer Skills: Session 40

Name of the session: _____

Name of the faculty member(s): _____

Date:_____   Time: _____   Duration:_____

Learning objective(s) of the session:

1. _____   2. _____

3. _____   4. _____

Teaching learning method(s):_____

REFLECTION

A. Please describe what happened during the session:

_____

_____

_____

_____

B. What did you learn from the session?

_____

_____

_____

_____

C. How will it help you become a better doctor in the future?

_____

_____

_____

_____

Sports and Extracurricular Activities

Total Time 22 Hours

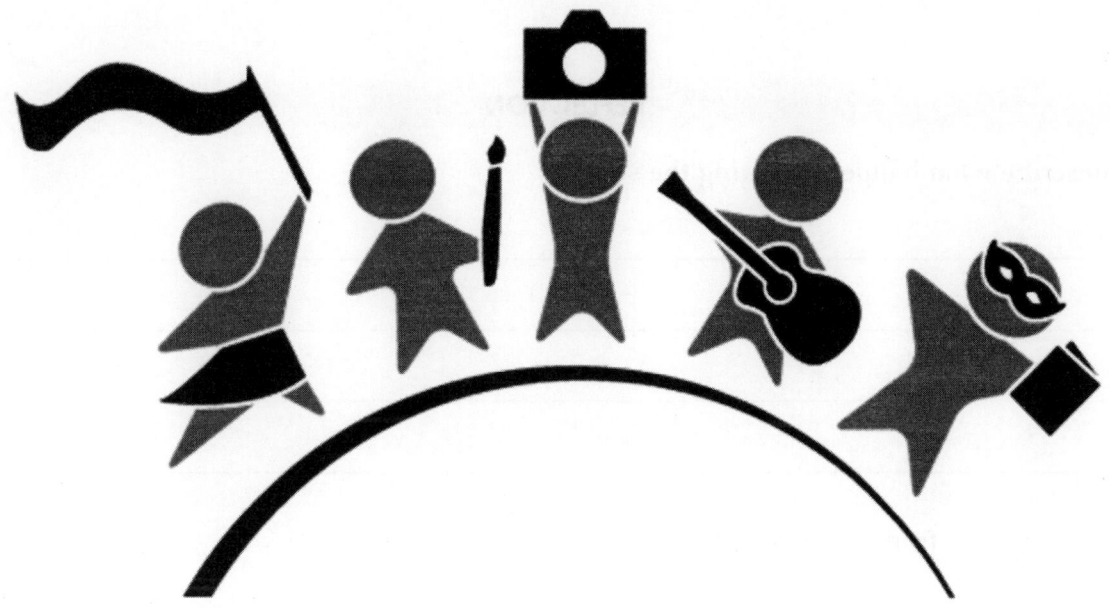

Sports and Extracurricular Activities: Session 1

Name of the session: _____

Name of the faculty member(s): _____

Date:_____   Time: _____   Duration:_____

Learning objective(s) of the session:

1. _____   2. _____

3. _____   4. _____

Teaching learning method(s):_____

REFLECTION

A. Please describe what happened during the session:

_____

_____

_____

_____

B. What did you learn from the session?

_____

_____

_____

_____

C. How will it help you become a better doctor in the future?

_____

_____

_____

_____

Sports and Extracurricular Activities: Session 2

Name of the session: _____

Name of the faculty member(s): _____

Date:_____   Time: _____   Duration:_____

Learning objective(s) of the session:

1. _____   2. _____

3. _____   4. _____

Teaching learning method(s):_____

REFLECTION

A. Please describe what happened during the session:

_____

_____

_____

_____

B. What did you learn from the session?

_____

_____

_____

_____

C. How will it help you become a better doctor in the future?

_____

_____

_____

Sports and Extracurricular Activities: Session 3

Name of the session: _____

Name of the faculty member(s): _____

Date:_____   Time: _____   Duration:_____

Learning objective(s) of the session:

1. _____   2. _____

3. _____   4. _____

Teaching learning method(s):_____

REFLECTION

A. Please describe what happened during the session:

_____

_____

_____

_____

B. What did you learn from the session?

_____

_____

_____

_____

C. How will it help you become a better doctor in the future?

_____

_____

_____

_____

Sports and Extracurricular Activities: Session 4

Name of the session: _____

Name of the faculty member(s): _____

Date:_____   Time: _____   Duration:_____

Learning objective(s) of the session:

1. _____   2. _____

3. _____   4. _____

Teaching learning method(s):_____

REFLECTION

A. Please describe what happened during the session:

_____

_____

_____

_____

B. What did you learn from the session?

_____

_____

_____

C. How will it help you become a better doctor in the future?

_____

_____

_____

Sports and Extracurricular Activities: Session 5

Name of the session: _____

Name of the faculty member(s): _____

Date:_____   Time: _____   Duration:_____

Learning objective(s) of the session:

1. _____   2. _____

3. _____   4. _____

Teaching learning method(s):_____

REFLECTION

A. Please describe what happened during the session:

_____

_____

_____

_____

B. What did you learn from the session?

_____

_____

_____

_____

C. How will it help you become a better doctor in the future?

_____

_____

_____

_____

Sports and Extracurricular Activities: Session 6

Name of the session: _____

Name of the faculty member(s): _____

Date:_____   Time: _____   Duration:_____

Learning objective(s) of the session:

1. _____   2. _____

3. _____   4. _____

Teaching learning method(s):_____

REFLECTION

A. Please describe what happened during the session:

_____

_____

_____

_____

B. What did you learn from the session?

_____

_____

_____

_____

C. How will it help you become a better doctor in the future?

_____

_____

_____

_____

Sports and Extracurricular Activities: Session 7

Name of the session: _____

Name of the faculty member(s): _____

Date:_____   Time: _____   Duration:_____

Learning objective(s) of the session:

1. _____   2. _____

3. _____   4. _____

Teaching learning method(s):_____

REFLECTION

A. Please describe what happened during the session:

_____

_____

_____

_____

B. What did you learn from the session?

_____

_____

_____

_____

C. How will it help you become a better doctor in the future?

_____

_____

_____

Sports and Extracurricular Activities: Session 8

Name of the session: _____

Name of the faculty member(s): _____

Date:_____   Time: _____   Duration:_____

Learning objective(s) of the session:

1. _____   2. _____

3. _____   4. _____

Teaching learning method(s):_____

REFLECTION

A. Please describe what happened during the session:

_____

_____

_____

_____

B. What did you learn from the session?

_____

_____

_____

_____

C. How will it help you become a better doctor in the future?

_____

_____

_____

_____

Sports and Extracurricular Activities: Session 9

Name of the session: _____

Name of the faculty member(s): _____

Date:_____   Time: _____   Duration:_____

Learning objective(s) of the session:

1. _____   2. _____

3. _____   4. _____

Teaching learning method(s):_____

REFLECTION

A. Please describe what happened during the session:

_____

_____

_____

_____

B. What did you learn from the session?

_____

_____

_____

_____

C. How will it help you become a better doctor in the future?

_____

_____

_____

_____

Sports and Extracurricular Activities: Session 10

Name of the session: _____

Name of the faculty member(s): _____

Date:_____   Time: _____   Duration:_____

Learning objective(s) of the session:

1. _____   2. _____

3. _____   4. _____

Teaching learning method(s):_____

REFLECTION

A. Please describe what happened during the session:

_____

_____

_____

_____

B. What did you learn from the session?

_____

_____

_____

C. How will it help you become a better doctor in the future?

_____

_____

_____

_____

Sports and Extracurricular Activities: Session 11

Name of the session: _____

Name of the faculty member(s): _____

Date:_____   Time:_____   Duration:_____

Learning objective(s) of the session:

1. _____   2. _____

3. _____   4. _____

Teaching learning method(s):_____

REFLECTION

A. Please describe what happened during the session:

_____

_____

_____

_____

B. What did you learn from the session?

_____

_____

_____

_____

C. How will it help you become a better doctor in the future?

_____

_____

_____

_____

Sports and Extracurricular Activities: Session 12

Name of the session: _____

Name of the faculty member(s): _____

Date:_____   Time: _____   Duration:_____

Learning objective(s) of the session:

1. _____   2. _____

3. _____   4. _____

Teaching learning method(s):_____

REFLECTION

A. Please describe what happened during the session:

_____

_____

_____

_____

B. What did you learn from the session?

_____

_____

_____

_____

C. How will it help you become a better doctor in the future?

_____

_____

_____

Sports and Extracurricular Activities: Session 13

Name of the session: _____

Name of the faculty member(s): _____

Date: _____ Time: _____ Duration: _____

Learning objective(s) of the session:

1. _____ 2. _____

3. _____ 4. _____

Teaching learning method(s): _____

REFLECTION

A. Please describe what happened during the session:

_____

_____

_____

_____

B. What did you learn from the session?

_____

_____

_____

_____

C. How will it help you become a better doctor in the future?

_____

_____

_____

_____

Sports and Extracurricular Activities: Session 14

Name of the session: _____

Name of the faculty member(s): _____

Date:_____   Time: _____   Duration:_____

Learning objective(s) of the session:

1. _____   2. _____

3. _____   4. _____

Teaching learning method(s):_____

REFLECTION

A. Please describe what happened during the session:

_____

_____

_____

_____

B. What did you learn from the session?

_____

_____

_____

_____

C. How will it help you become a better doctor in the future?

_____

_____

_____

_____

Sports and Extracurricular Activities: Session 15

Name of the session: _____

Name of the faculty member(s): _____

Date:_____   Time:_____   Duration:_____

Learning objective(s) of the session:

1. _____   2. _____

3. _____   4. _____

Teaching learning method(s):_____

REFLECTION

A. Please describe what happened during the session:

_____

_____

_____

_____

B. What did you learn from the session?

_____

_____

_____

C. How will it help you become a better doctor in the future?

_____

_____

_____

_____

Sports and Extracurricular Activities: Session 16

Name of the session: _____

Name of the faculty member(s): _____

Date:_____   Time:_____   Duration:_____

Learning objective(s) of the session:

1. _____   2. _____

3. _____   4. _____

Teaching learning method(s):_____

REFLECTION

A. Please describe what happened during the session:

_____

_____

_____

_____

B. What did you learn from the session?

_____

_____

_____

_____

C. How will it help you become a better doctor in the future?

_____

_____

_____

_____

Sports and Extracurricular Activities: Session 17

Name of the session: _____

Name of the faculty member(s): _____

Date: _____   Time: _____   Duration: _____

Learning objective(s) of the session:

1. _____   2. _____

3. _____   4. _____

Teaching learning method(s): _____

REFLECTION

A. Please describe what happened during the session:

_____

_____

_____

_____

B. What did you learn from the session?

_____

_____

_____

_____

C. How will it help you become a better doctor in the future?

_____

_____

_____

Sports and Extracurricular Activities: Session 18

Name of the session: _____

Name of the faculty member(s): _____

Date:_____ Time: _____ Duration:_____

Learning objective(s) of the session:

1. _____ 2. _____

3. _____ 4. _____

Teaching learning method(s):_____

REFLECTION

A. Please describe what happened during the session:

_____

_____

_____

_____

B. What did you learn from the session?

_____

_____

_____

_____

C. How will it help you become a better doctor in the future?

_____

_____

_____

_____

Sports and Extracurricular Activities: Session 19

Name of the session: _____

Name of the faculty member(s): _____

Date:_____   Time: _____   Duration:_____

Learning objective(s) of the session:

1. _____   2. _____

3. _____   4. _____

Teaching learning method(s):_____

REFLECTION

A. Please describe what happened during the session:

_____

_____

_____

_____

B. What did you learn from the session?

_____

_____

_____

_____

C. How will it help you become a better doctor in the future?

_____

_____

_____

_____

Sports and Extracurricular Activities: Session 20

Name of the session: _____

Name of the faculty member(s): _____

Date:_____   Time: _____   Duration:_____

Learning objective(s) of the session:

1. _____   2. _____

3. _____   4. _____

Teaching learning method(s):_____

REFLECTION

A. Please describe what happened during the session:

_____

_____

_____

_____

B. What did you learn from the session?

_____

_____

_____

_____

C. How will it help you become a better doctor in the future?

_____

_____

_____

_____

Sports and Extracurricular Activities: Session 21

Name of the session: _____

Name of the faculty member(s): _____

Date: _____   Time: _____   Duration: _____

Learning objective(s) of the session:

1. _____   2. _____

3. _____   4. _____

Teaching learning method(s): _____

REFLECTION

A. Please describe what happened during the session:

_____

_____

_____

_____

B. What did you learn from the session?

_____

_____

_____

_____

C. How will it help you become a better doctor in the future?

_____

_____

_____

_____

Sports and Extracurricular Activities: Session 22

Name of the session: _____

Name of the faculty member(s): _____

Date:_____   Time: _____   Duration:_____

Learning objective(s) of the session:

1. _____   2. _____

3. _____   4. _____

Teaching learning method(s):_____

REFLECTION

A. Please describe what happened during the session:

_____

_____

_____

_____

B. What did you learn from the session?

_____

_____

_____

C. How will it help you become a better doctor in the future?

_____

_____

_____

_____